# 7-DAY
# PHONE DETOX

# ☐ Turn off all push notifications

- Let's be honest, we don't need to know when anyone likes or comments on our social media posts. We don't need to know each time we get a new email. We don't need to know each news story when it breaks (talk about depressing!).
- Let's say you get 10 notifications per day (that's being conservative!) and each one distracts you for 5 minutes, that's almost an hour per day wasted!
- It's time to turn off ALL of your notifications. How to do this will vary by phone but I challenge you to go do this right after reading this.

# HOW DO YOU FEEL?

# Unfollow Accounts That Make You Feel Bad About Yourself

- If you follow people that you think are inspiring but when you really think about it they just make you feel bad about yourself, unfollow them!
- If an account makes you feel like you don't make enough money, don't have the ideal body, don't have the perfect kids or house unfollow them!

# HOW DO YOU FEEL?

# ☐ Limit Your Hours on Social Media

- Establish your own rules for your social media (or phone in general) use. These can vary based on your lifestyle, a good starting point is never before 10 AM and never after 8 PM.
- You could set the alarm on your phone to remind you to turn off or activate your do not disturb feature at these times. No excuses, turn them off!

# HOW DO YOU FEEL?

☐ # Delete Apps You Never Use

- This is an easy day! Go through your phone and delete the apps you never use! They are always glaring back at you when you look at your phone. Clean them off and clean it up!

# HOW DO YOU FEEL?

## DAY 5

# ☐ Read a Book Instead of Scrolling

- It's INSANE how much time we spend scrolling through social media. We would all be completely shocked if we truly knew the amount of time we have wasted. Sure, some of it isn't wasted but we all get sucked in and then before you know it 10 minutes···or 1 hour goes by and we're still scrolling!
- Pick up a physical book (try to resist reading one on your phone!) and start reading. Learn something new or just zone out with your favorite non-fiction book.

# HOW DO YOU FEEL?

DAY 6

- [ ] # Create Memories without Posting Pictures on Social Media

- You can take pictures with your phone (if you insist!) but don't post them on social media. Instead, ENJOY the moment. Take in everything that is happening without feeling the need to immediately post on Instagram and Facebook.

# HOW DO YOU FEEL?

# DAY 7

☐ Turn Off Your Phone for the Entire Day

- It's not as hard you might think! YOU CAN DO IT! Turn off your cell phone for an entire day and just be COMPLETELY in the moment. You've done it before cell phones, you can do it again.

# HOW DO YOU FEEL?

Good job!

# You did it!

# NOTES

# NOTES

NOTES

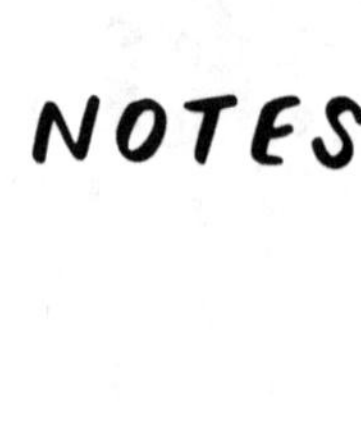

# NOTES

# NOTES

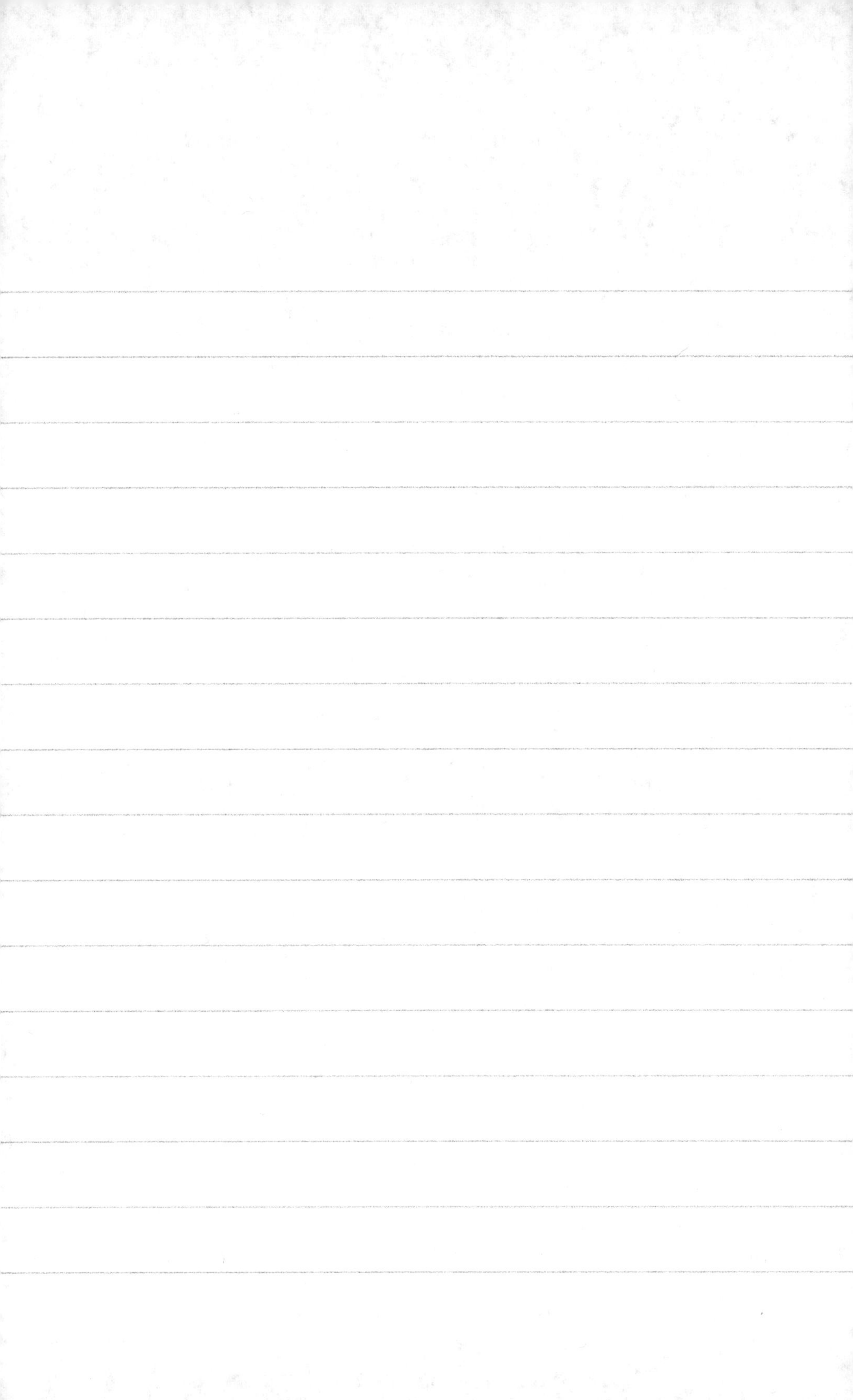

# NOTES

# NOTES

# NOTES

# NOTES

# NOTES

# NOTES

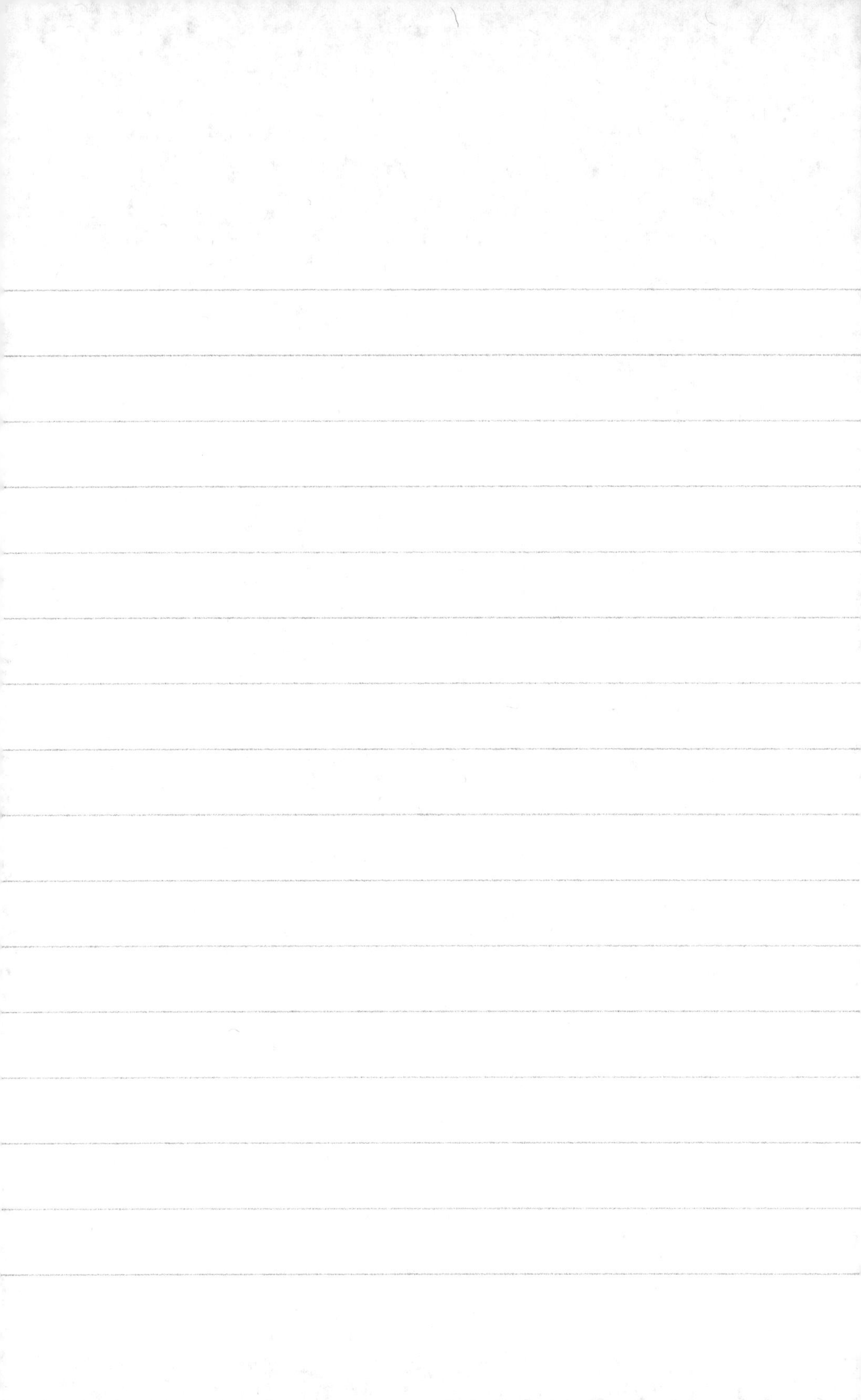

# NOTES

# NOTES

# NOTES

# NOTES

# NOTES

# NOTES

# NOTES

# NOTES

# NOTES

# NOTES

# NOTES

# NOTES

# NOTES

# NOTES

# NOTES

# NOTES

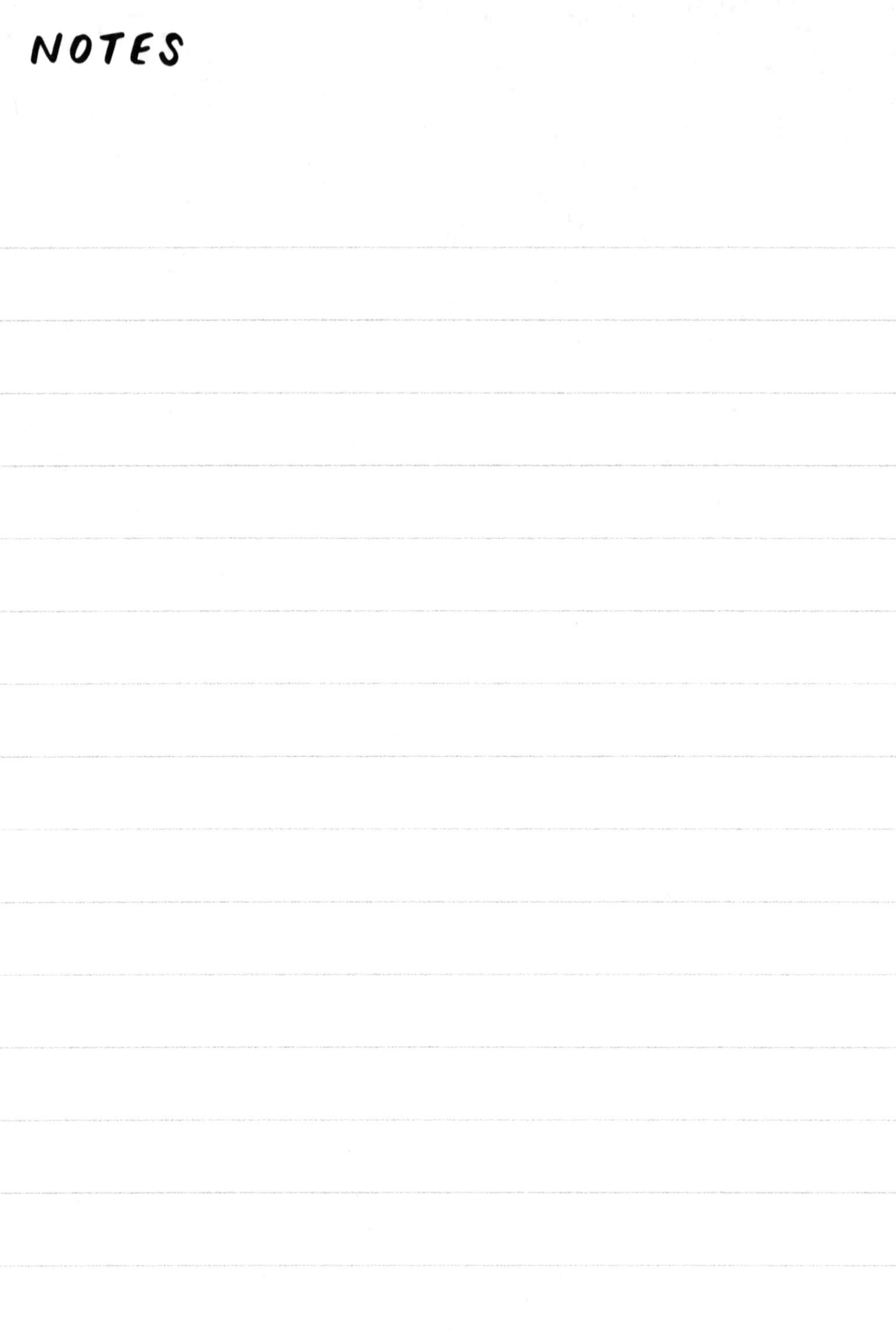

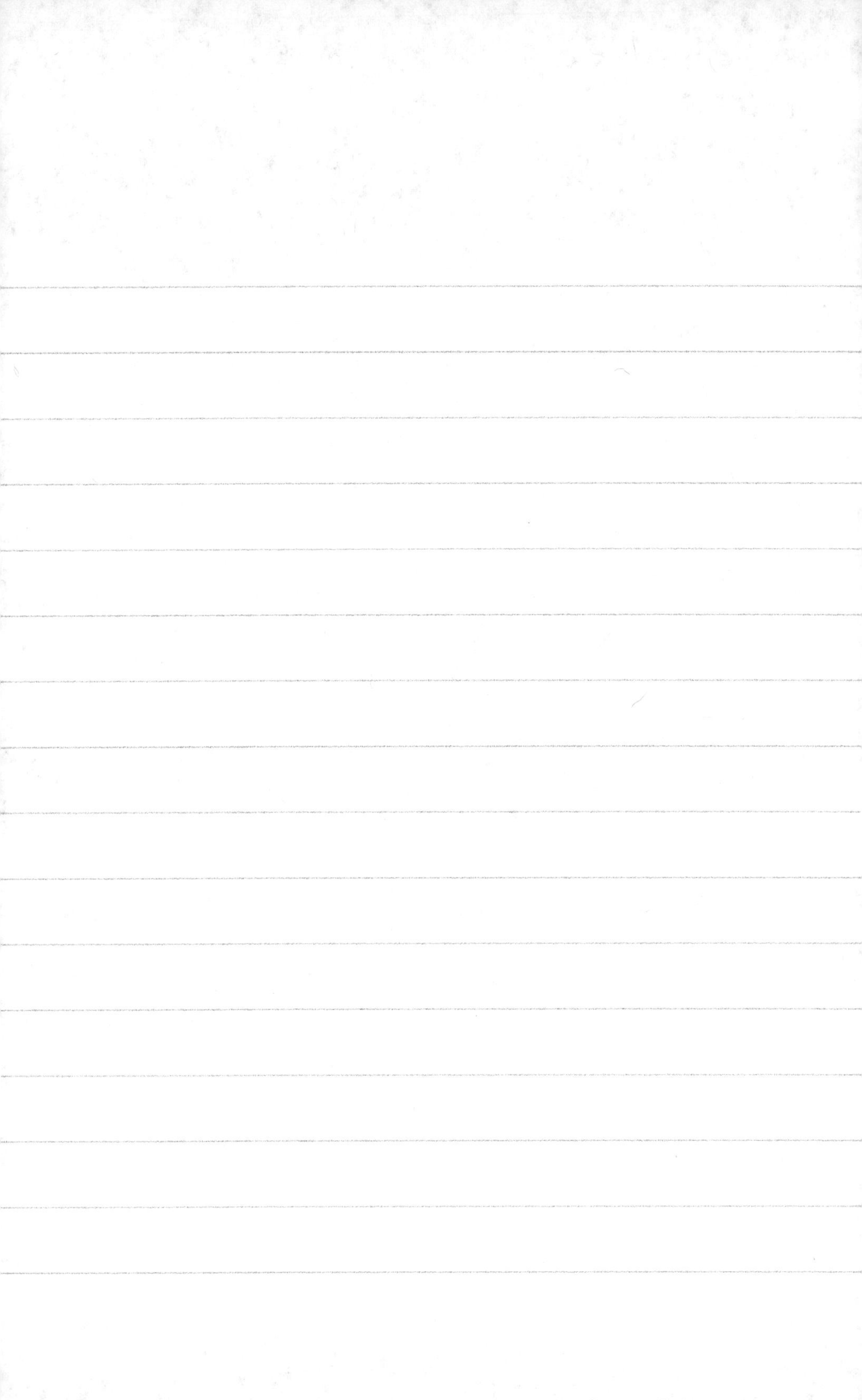

# NOTES

# NOTES

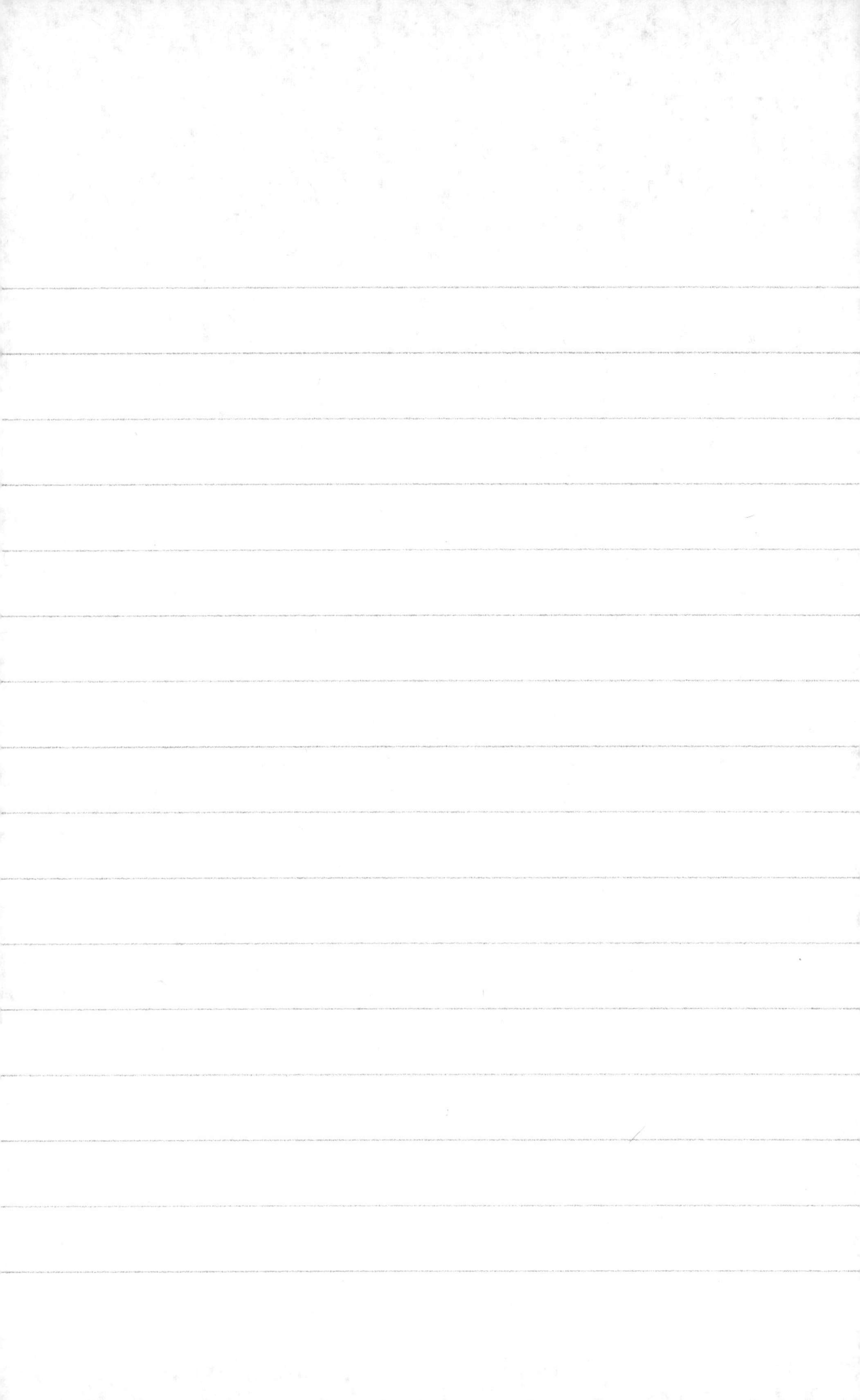

# NOTES

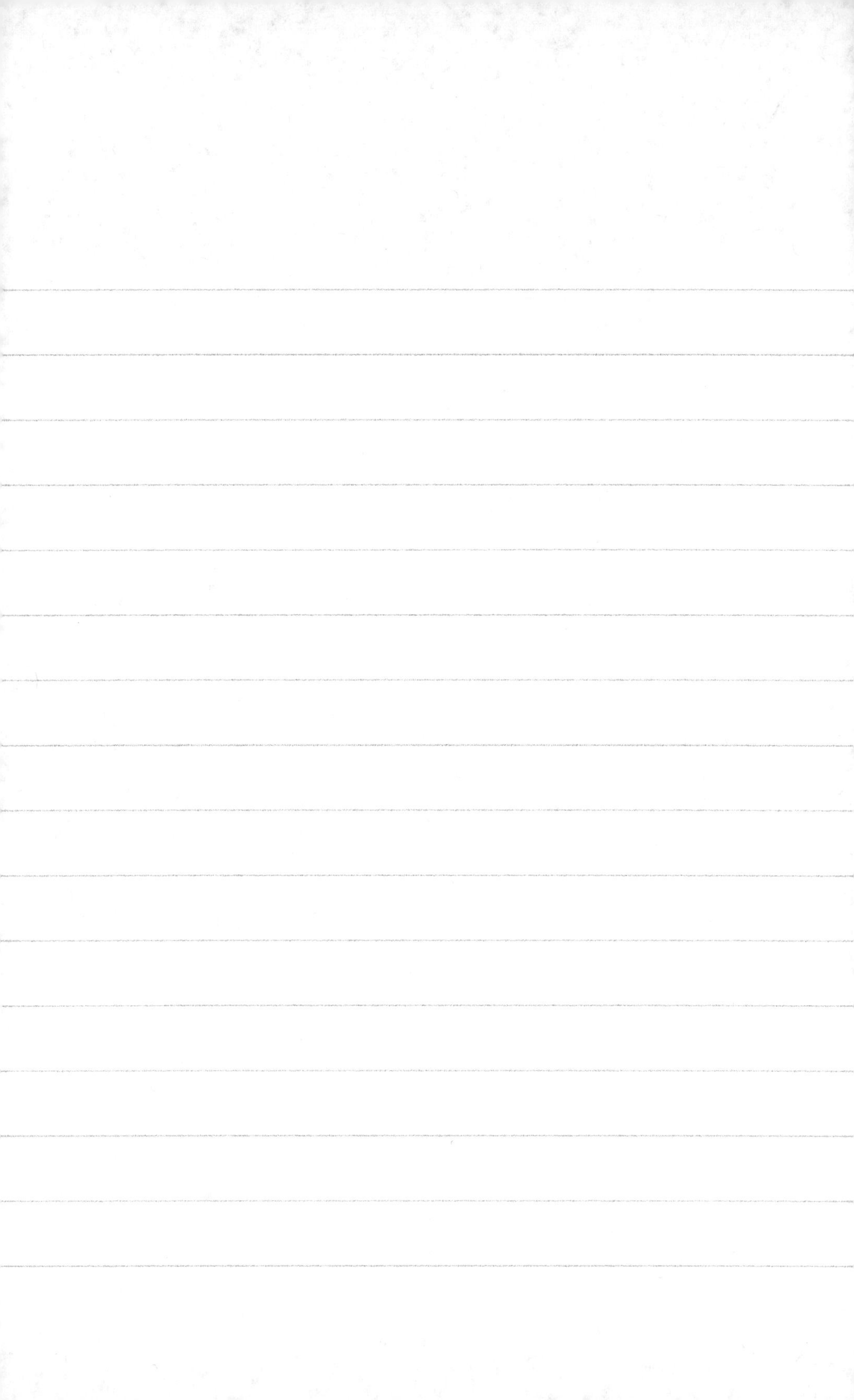

# NOTES

# NOTES

# NOTES

# NOTES

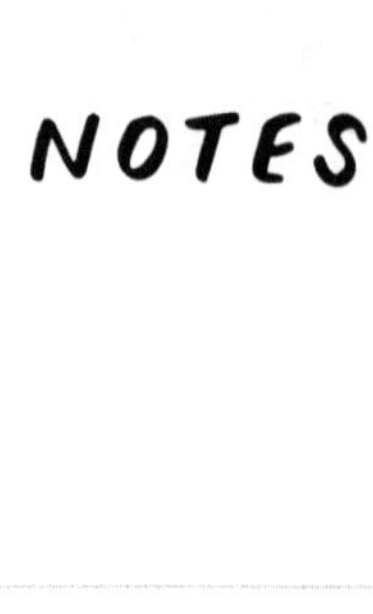
NOTES

# NOTES

# NOTES

# NOTES

# NOTES

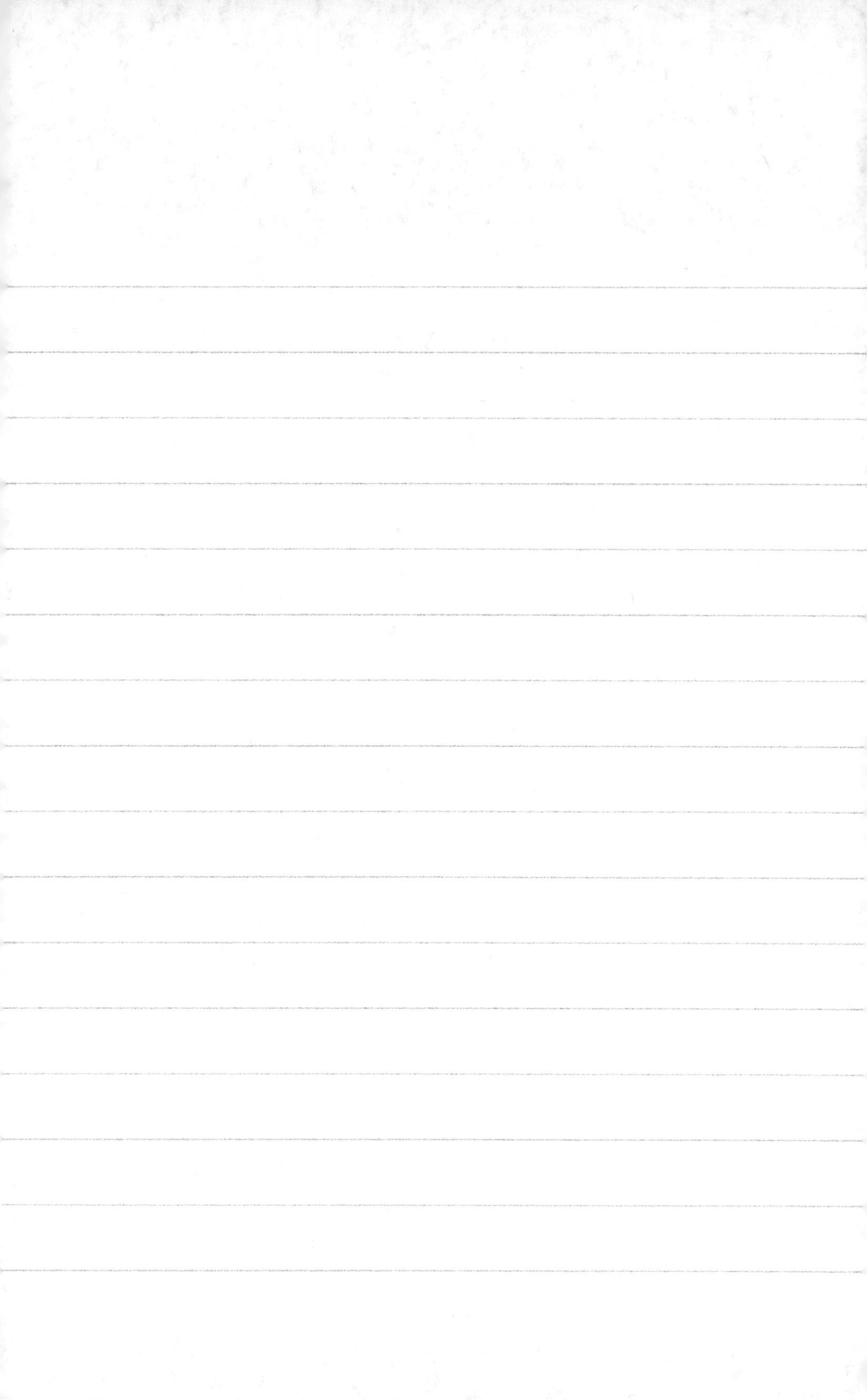

# NOTES

GOOD KARMA BOOKS